WHAT IN THE WORLD IS THE CORONAVIRUS?

MARTINA MARIE DOMINO

This book is dedicated to the greatest and most supportive mother and father anyone could ever have, Debra and Rudolph. Thanks for always pushing me to follow my dreams and always finish what I start.

This book is also for my sons: Jalen La'Mar, Jordan Tino, and Lloyd George III, and all of the children around the world that are having to cope with the changes and loss during this COVID-19 pandemic.

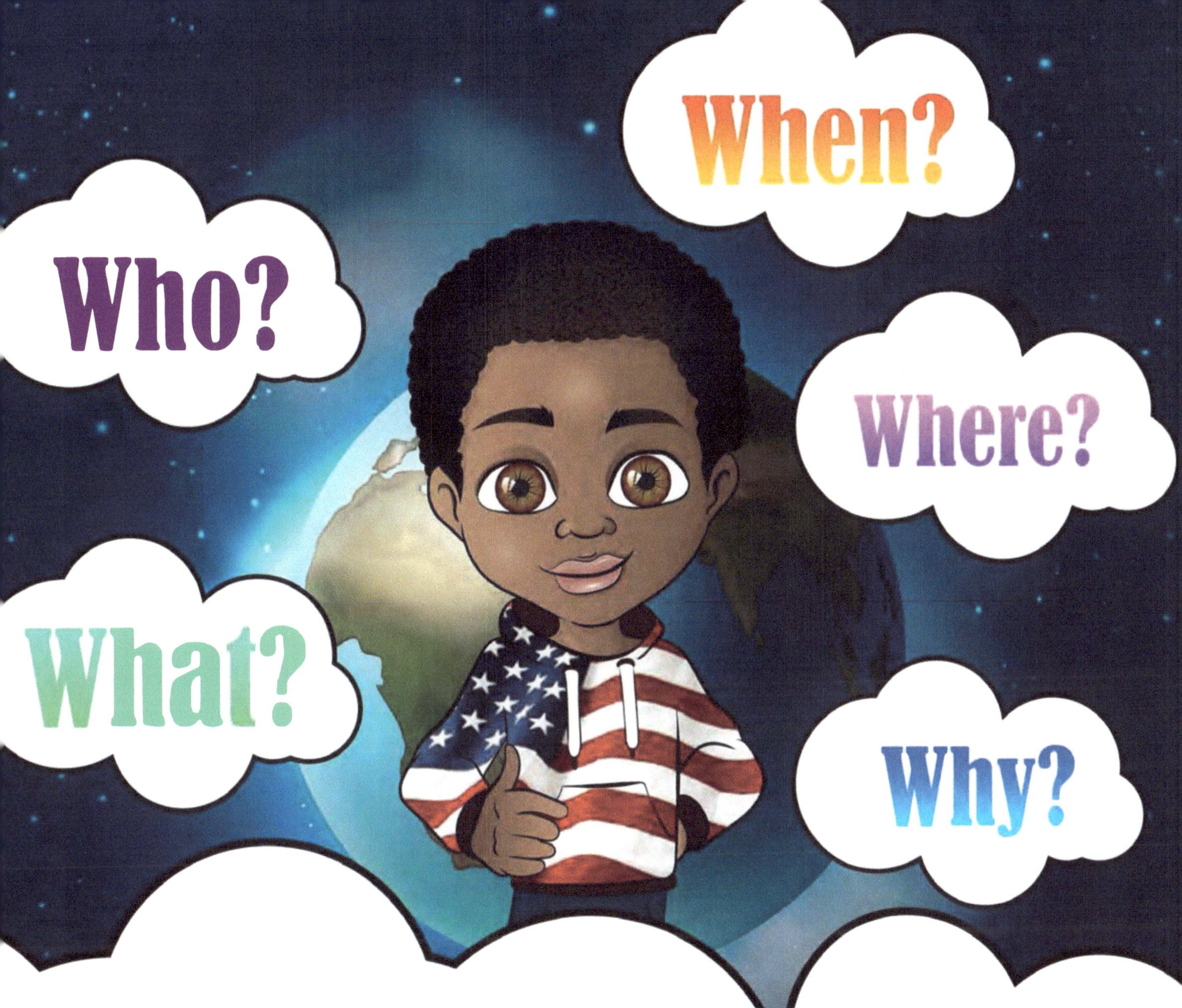

Hi there! My name is Jalen and I'm a W World Kid from the United States of America. W World Kids are from all over the world. We help kids just like you learn about different people, places, things, and more! We answer lots of questions about Who, What, When, Where and Why?! You're going to learn so many things with us. So, let's begin!

1

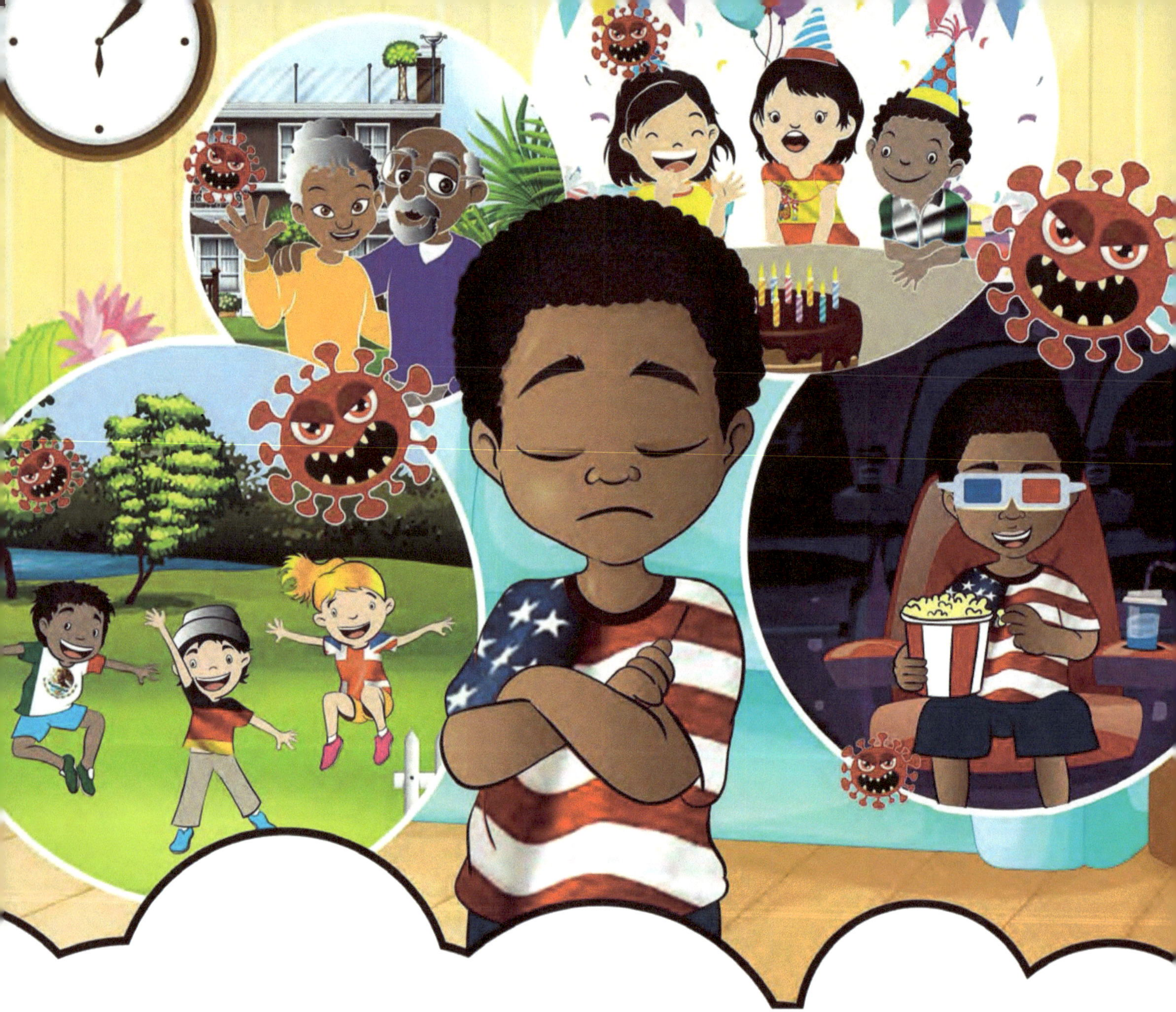

If you are a kid just like me, I know you may be thinking, "What in the world is the coronavirus?" We can't play outside with friends. We can't go and see our grandparents. We can't go to birthday parties.
We can't go to the movies.
All because of the coronavirus!

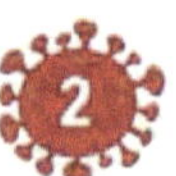

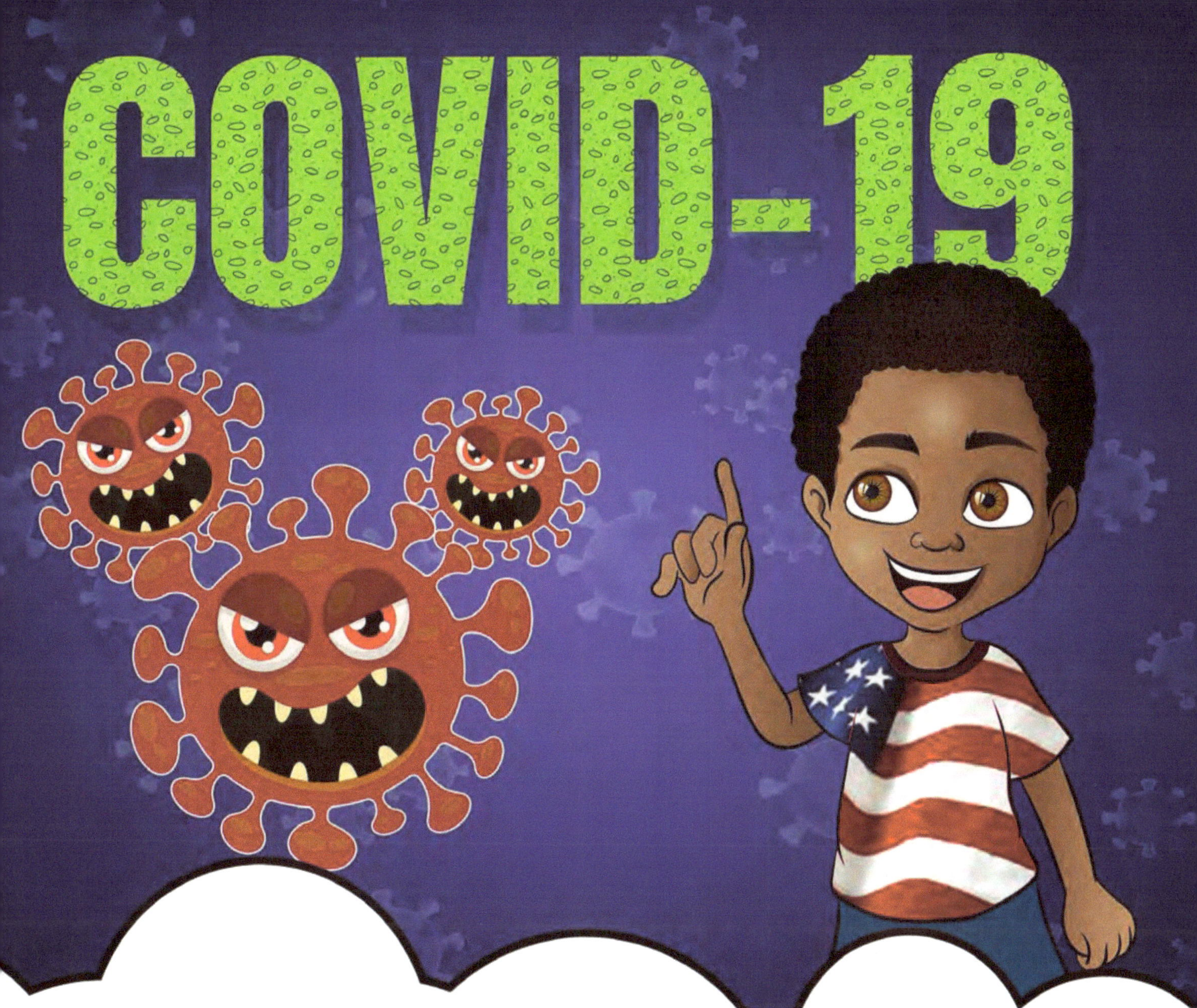

So, what is it? Well, I'm here to help you learn all about it.
The coronavirus is a virus. A virus is a germ that you can't see. If these germs get inside your body, they start a big germ party!
That is when you get sick with an illness called COVID-19.

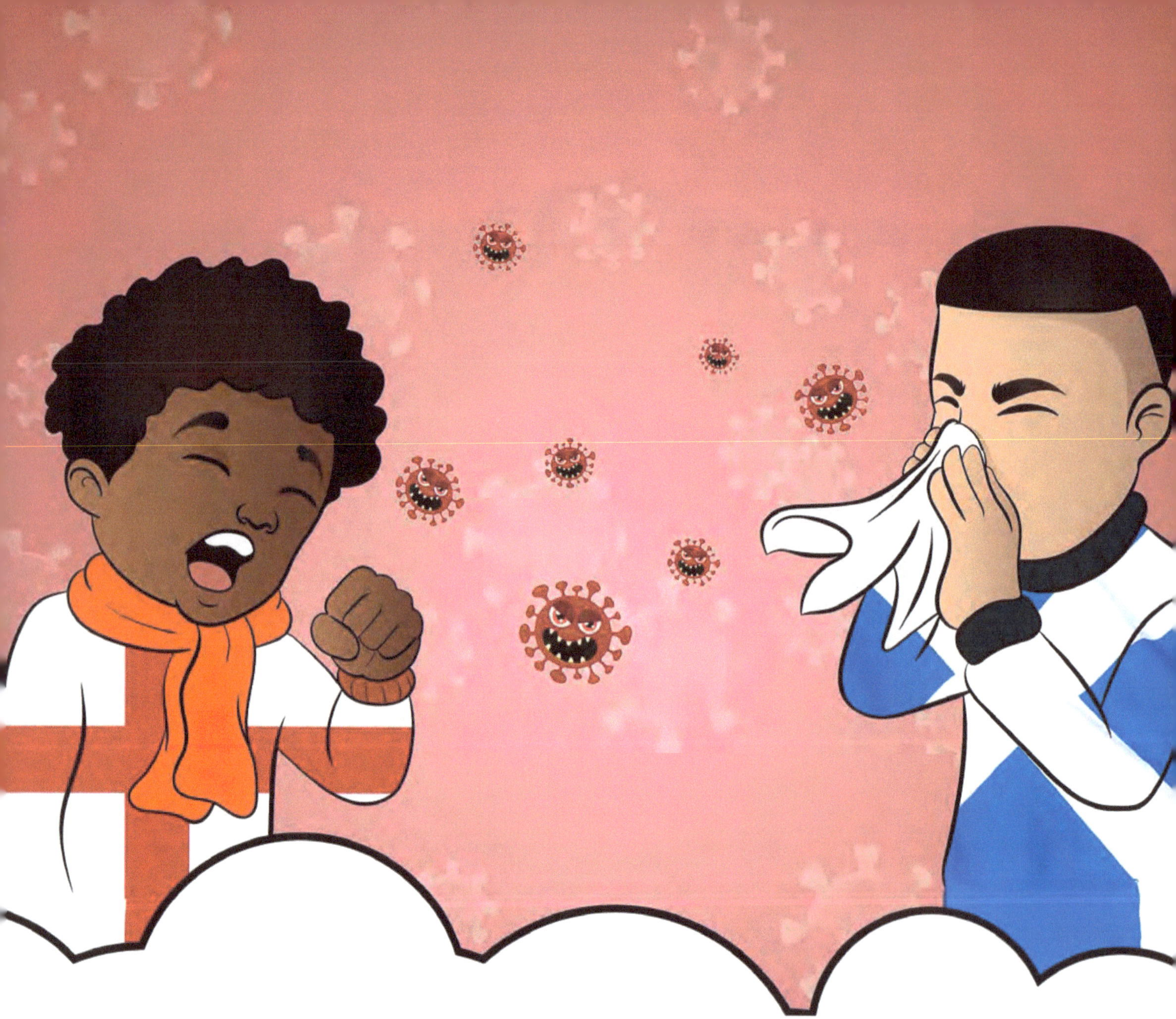

People catch this virus mostly when sick people cough, sneeze or talk.
The germs come out of their mouth or nose.
You can breathe it in without even seeing it!

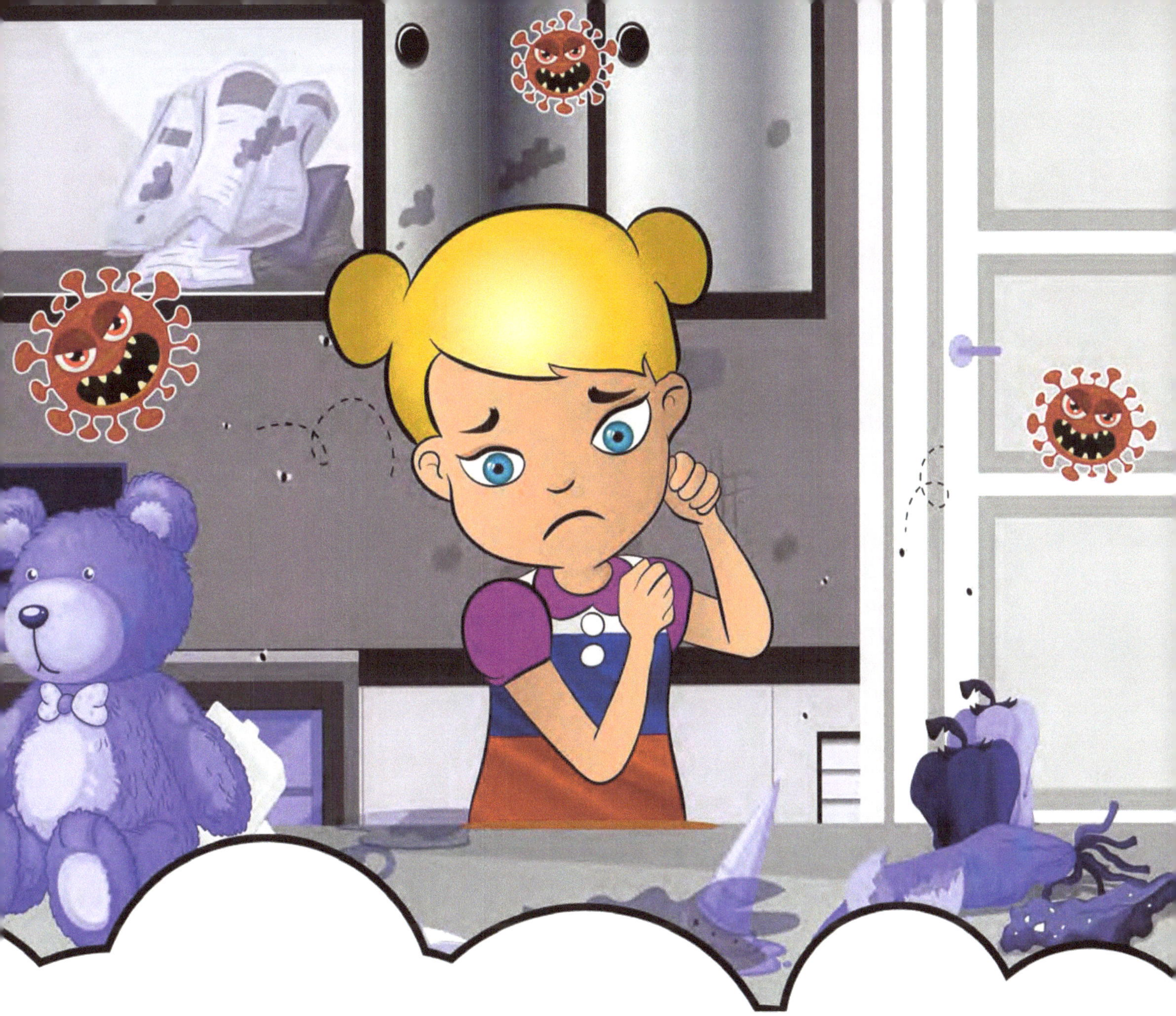

You can also catch the coronavirus by touching
a germy table or doorknob.
You can catch it by touching a germy toy too!

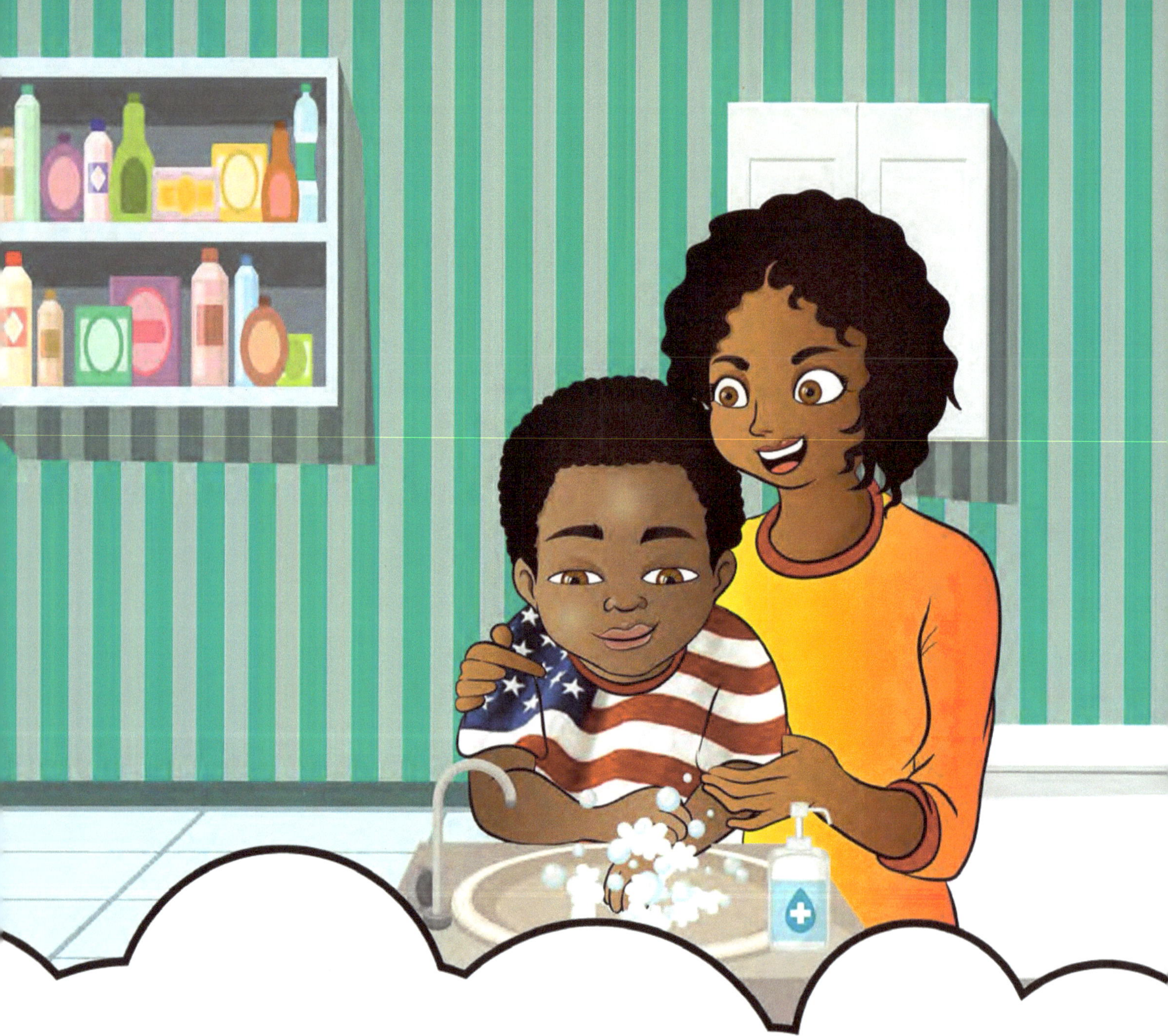

My mom says we need to wash our hands to keep the germs from getting inside of our bodies. When we wash our hands with soap and count to 20, we know they are all clean!

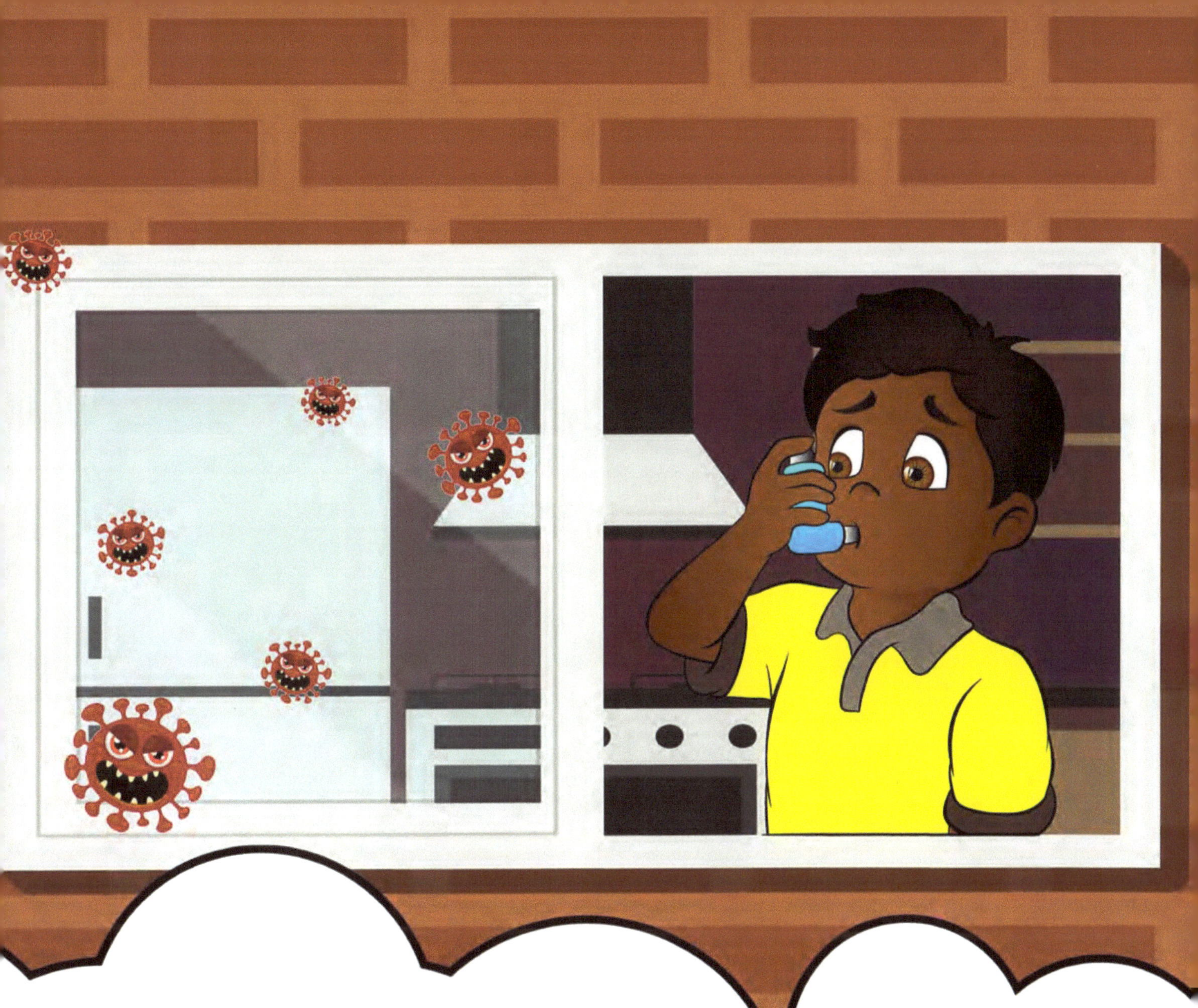

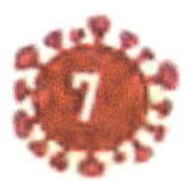

Most kids like you and I will not get very sick if we do catch the coronavirus.
My oldest brother has asthma, so he must be very careful not to catch it
because it would make it more difficult for him to breathe.
That is why it is important to stay inside so we do not make others sick.

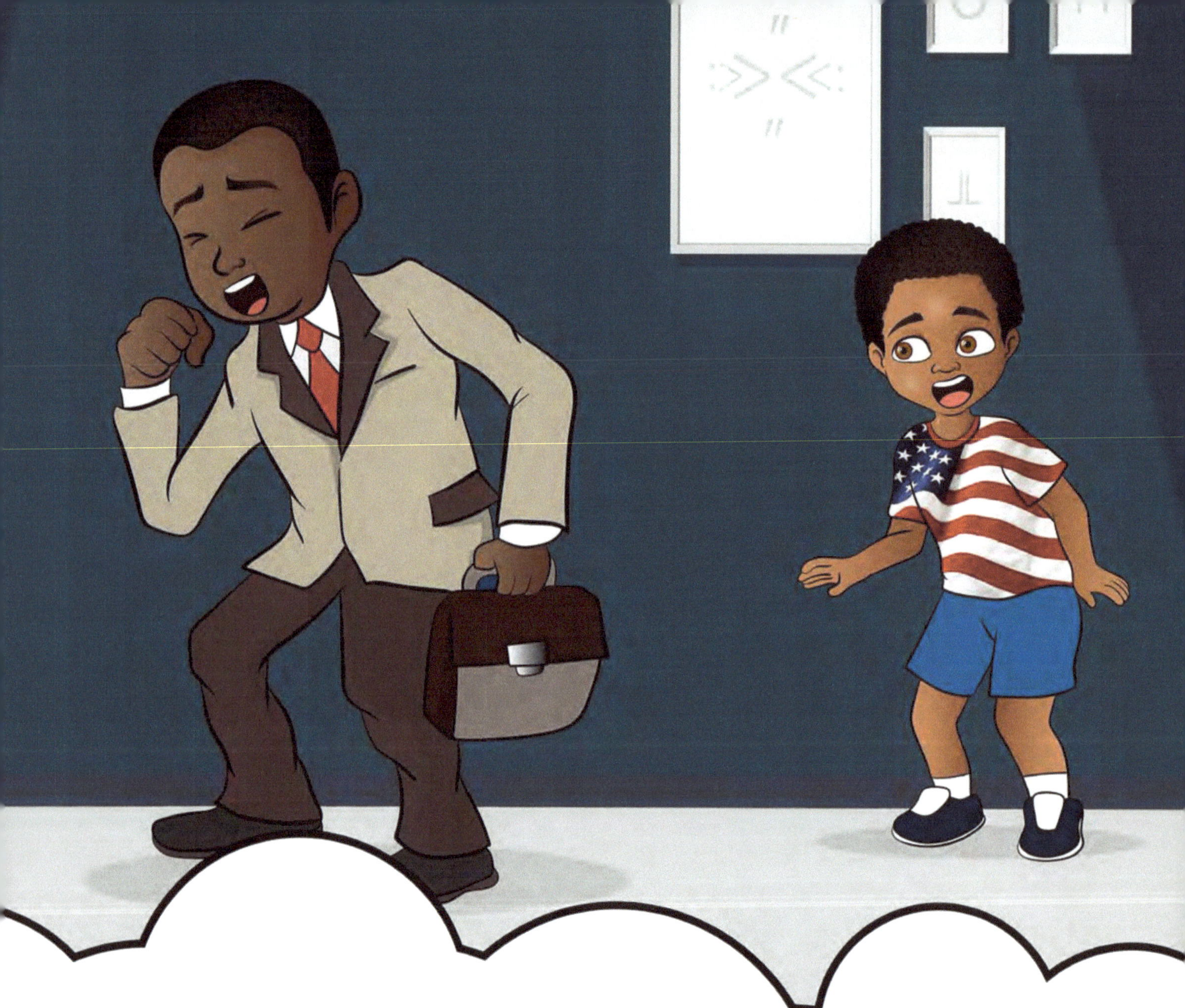

Last week, my dad seemed healthy. He said he did not feel sick and did not have a fever either. He had a small cough and was just sleepy. His manager sent him to take a rapid COVID-19 test. The results were positive for coronavirus! The doctor told him to isolate himself inside of the house for 14 days. Dad's body fought the coronavirus and now he's better.

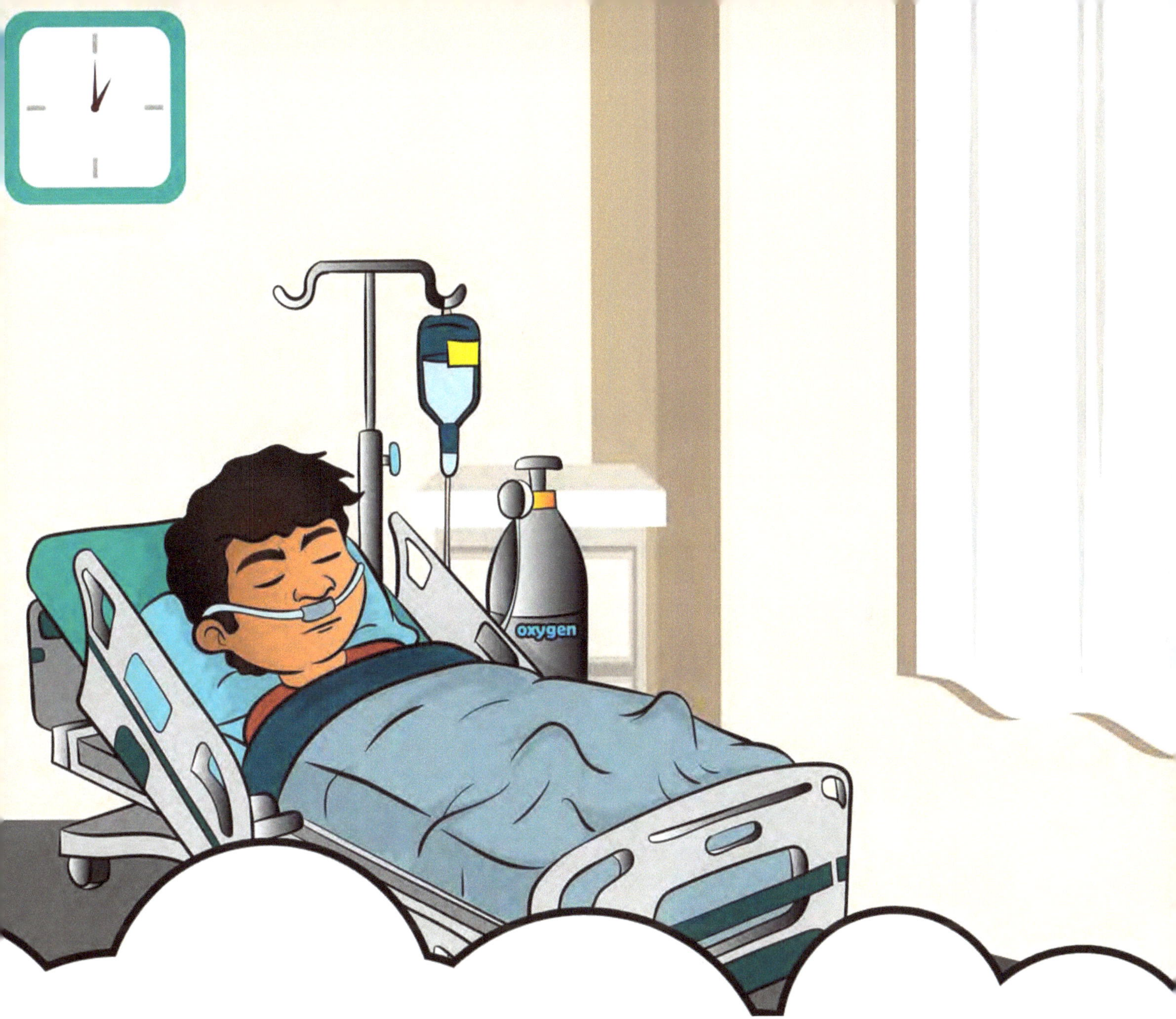

When Dad caught the coronavirus, Mom and I took a test too, but our results were negative. Other people are not so lucky. They can become very sick.

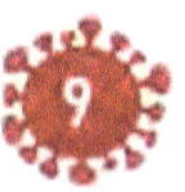

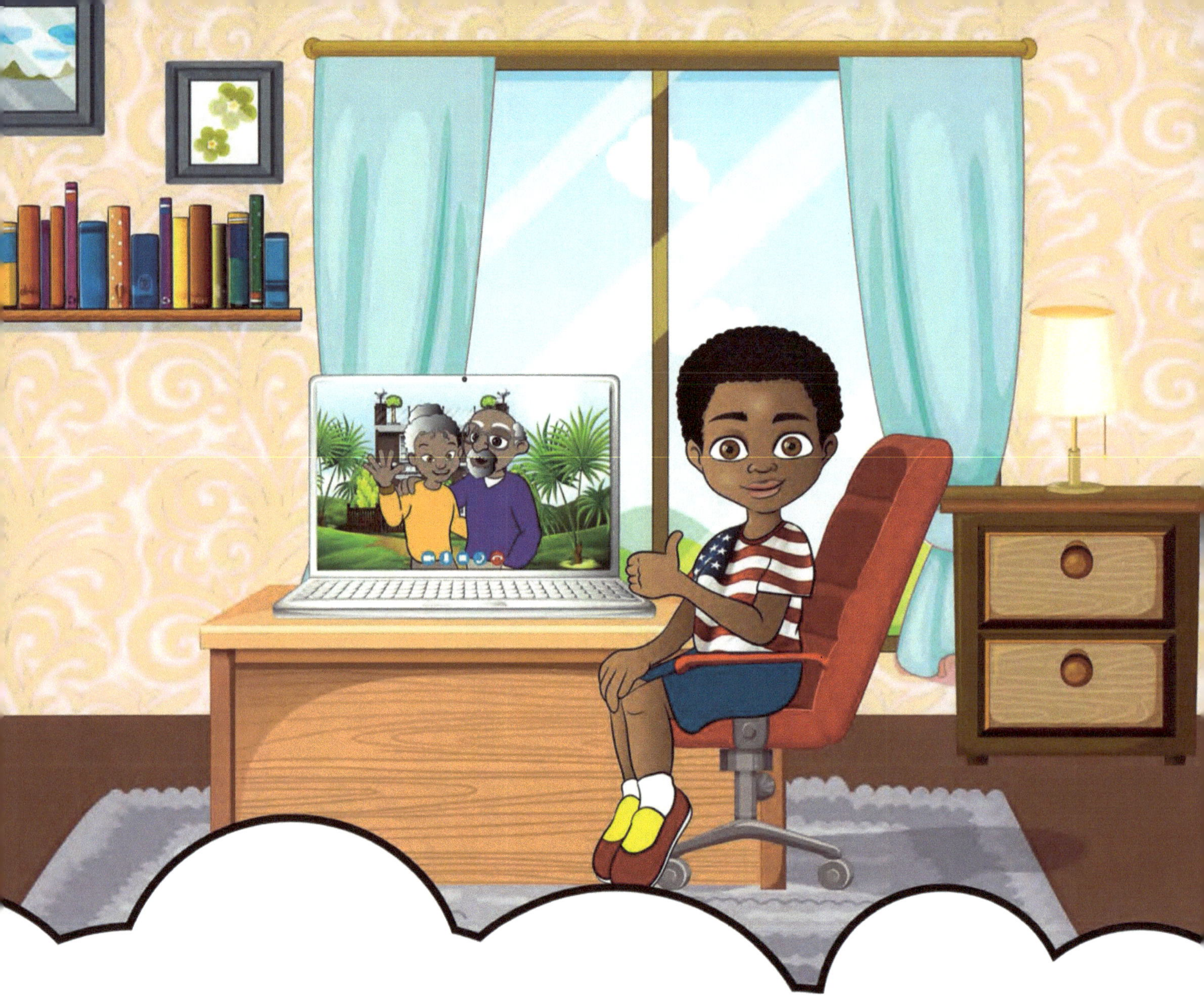

People like Grandma and Grandpa have a hard time fighting the coronavirus because their bodies are not as strong. Mom says we must practice social distancing and talk them on the phone or computer to see them and keep in touch.

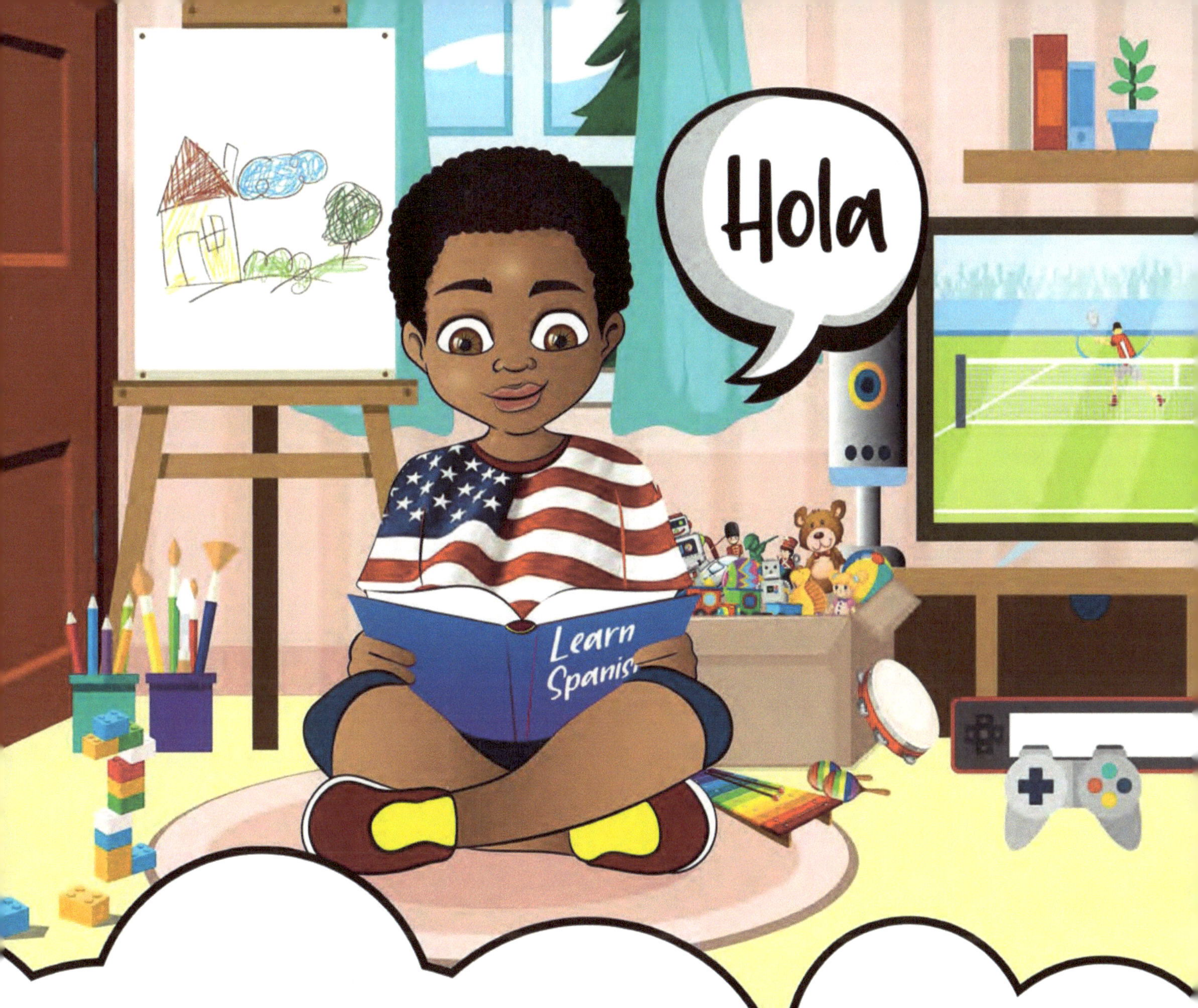

If you or someone in your home has to isolate because you or others are sick, you can do some of these fun activities to keep from being bored: puzzles, Legos, coloring, video games, reading, learn a foreign language or watch television.

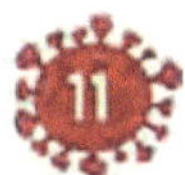

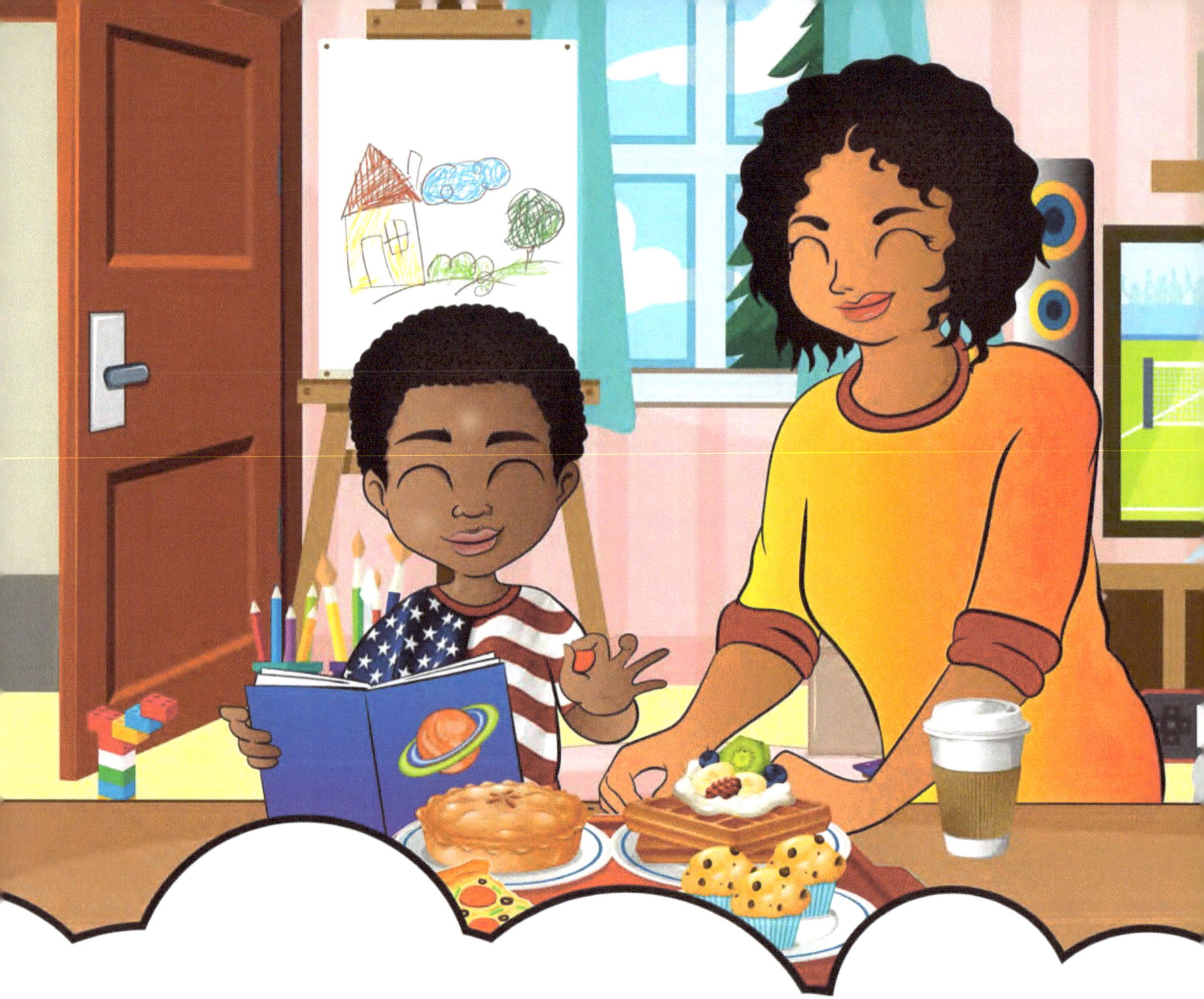

At first, I thought staying inside would not be fun, but it was actually kind of cool. My mom brought everyone breakfast, lunch, dinner, and snacks to their doors. I did not have to leave my room for anything because I had so many fun things to do. I just made the best of it!

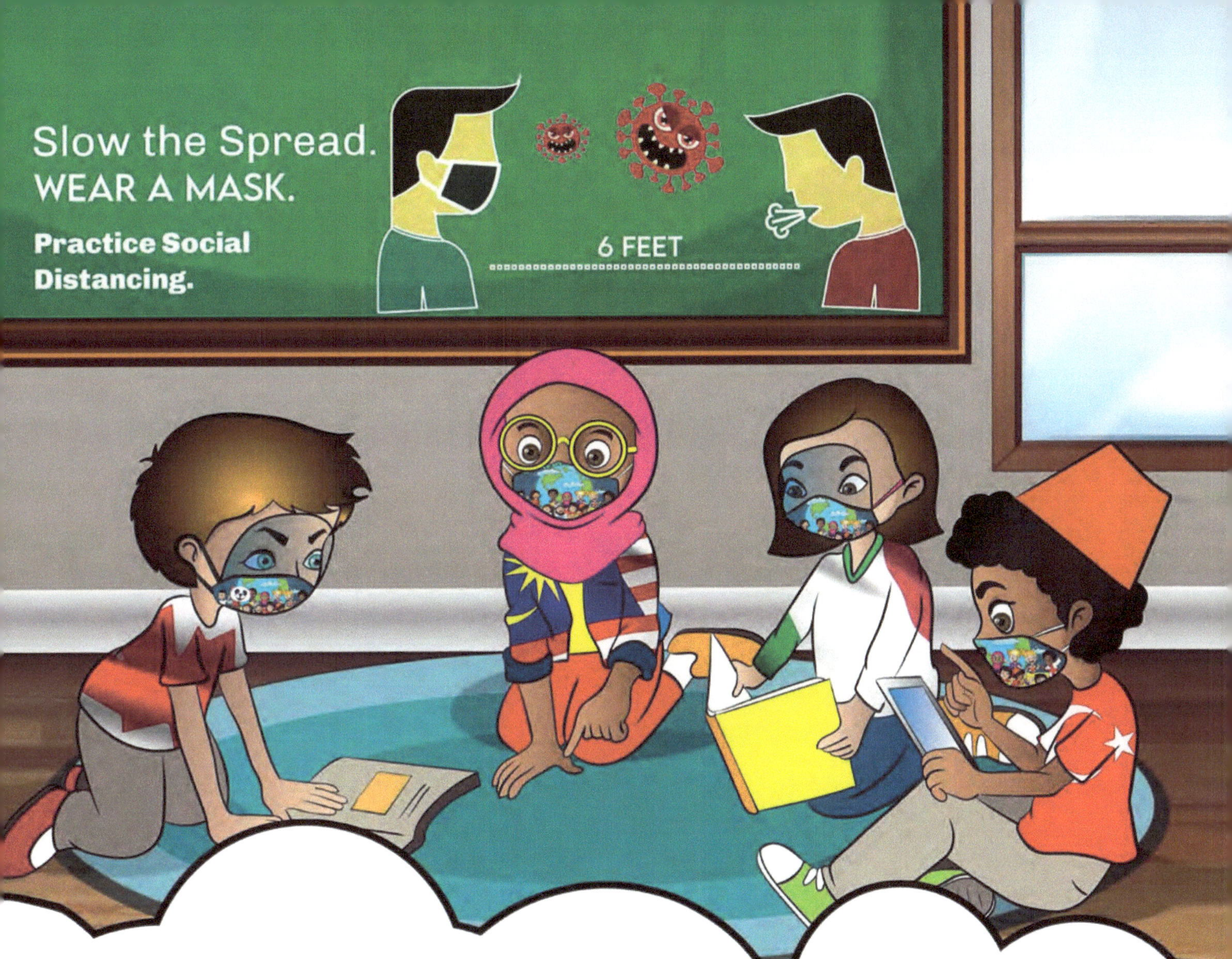

Once it's safe to roam freely again, do not forget to wear a mask.
Those coronavirus germs could flow right into your mouth or nose.
YUCK!

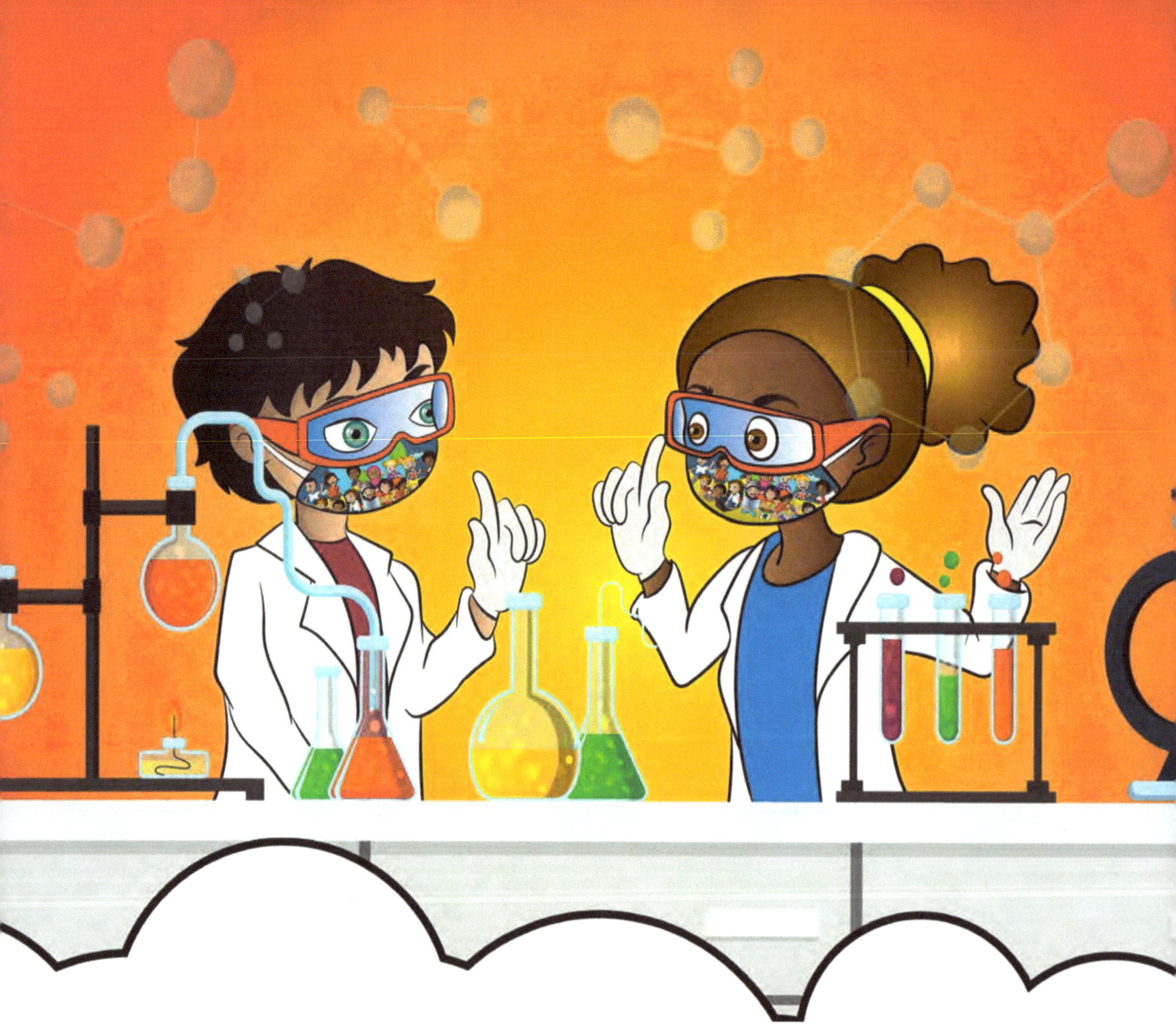

Doctors and scientists all around the world are actively working to develop the perfect vaccine for all of us. Though we haven't developed a PERFECT vaccine, the one we have is being given to doctors, nurses, and other first responders.

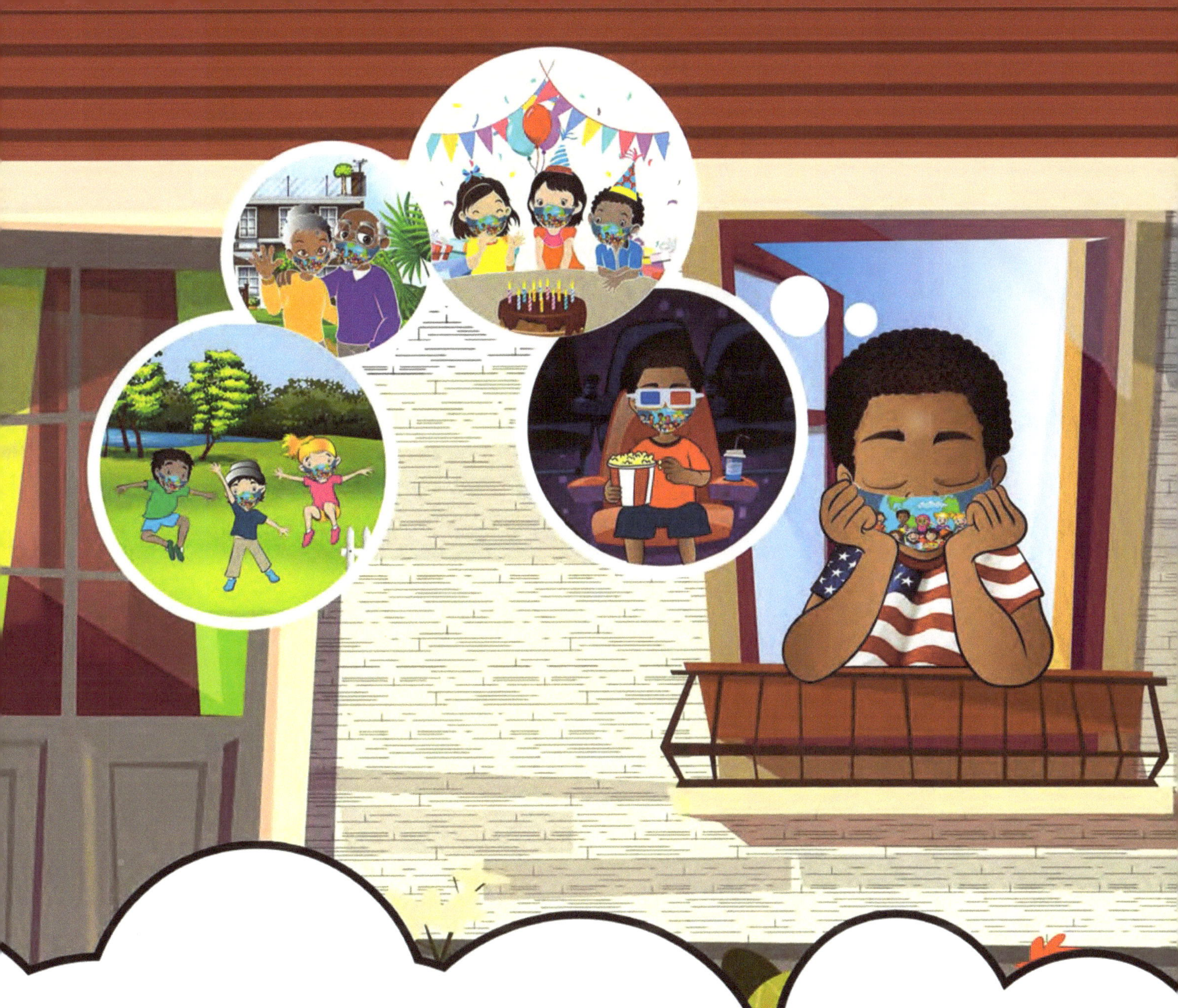

Once most people get vaccinated, we will once again be able to:
go play outside with friends, go and see our grandparents, go to birthday
parties and go to the movies. So, remember...be safe, stay inside, cover
your coughs and sneezes, do not touch your nose or mouth,
and wash your hands!

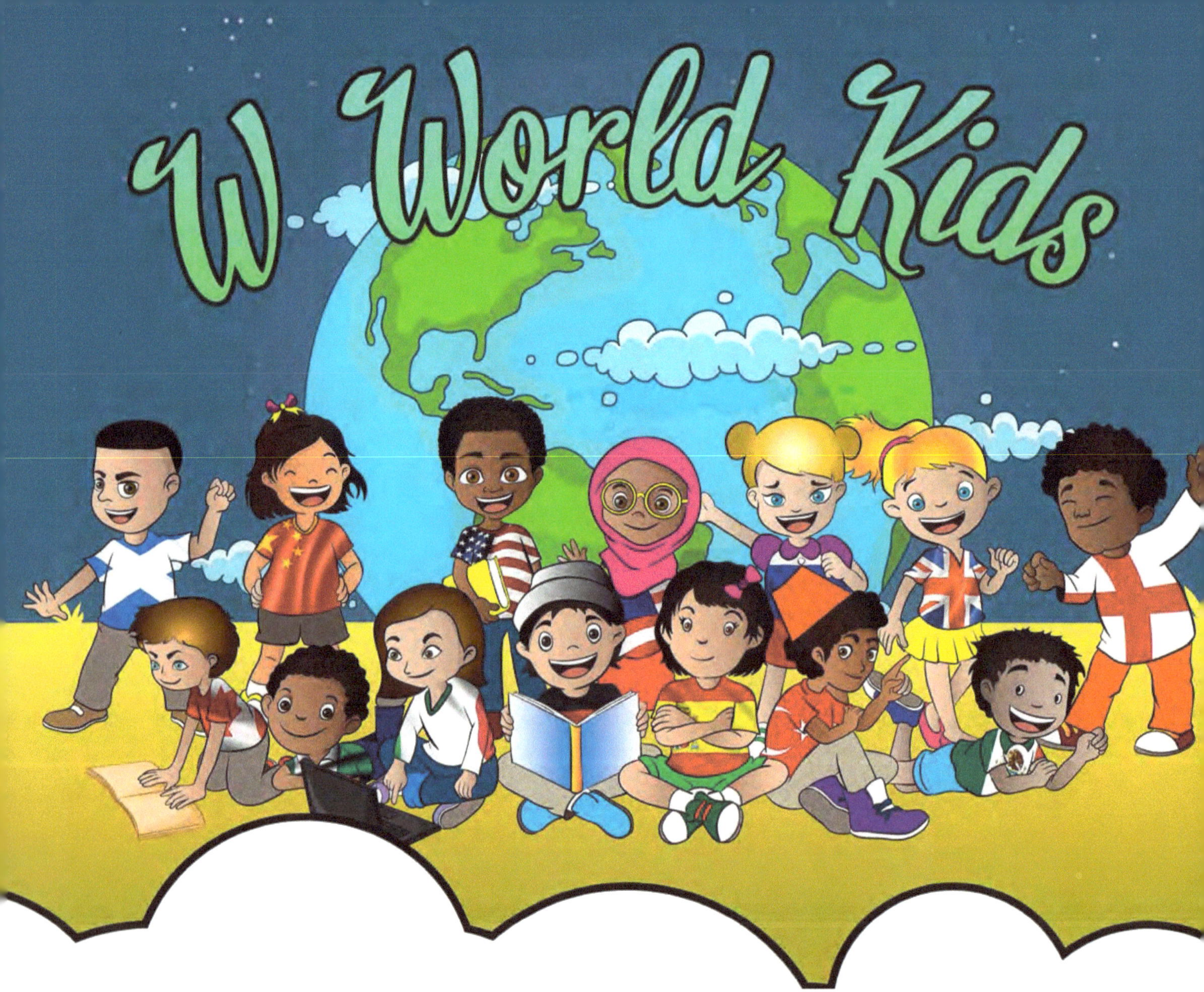

W World Kids

This will keep us all safe!
Until then, everyone in the world must keep
following the rules!
Us W World Kids too!

More information about the author:

Martina Domino's book, "What in the World is the
Coronavirus?" has received starred reviews and was a #1 New
Release in Children's Health on Amazon.com.

She was born and raised in Baton Rouge, Louisiana and received
her bachelor's and master's degree
from Southern University and A & M College.

When she is not writing, Martina spends most of her time
reading, traveling, snorkeling, zip-lining, shopping, and doing
anything else adventurous!

Being a New Orleans Saints sports fanatic since the age of four,
she watches football on Sunday afternoons!

Keep in touch with Martina via the web:
Website: https://www.martinadomino.com
Facebook: http://www.facebook.com/AuthorMartinaDomino
Instagram: https://instagram.com/authormartinadomino/

Don't forget to submit a review wherever your book
was purchased.

Also, help name a new character! He has a question mark
underneath him. Can you choose a name to match the country he
is from? Submit your entry on any of the social media accounts
listed above for a chance to win a W World Kids face mask!
Good Luck!

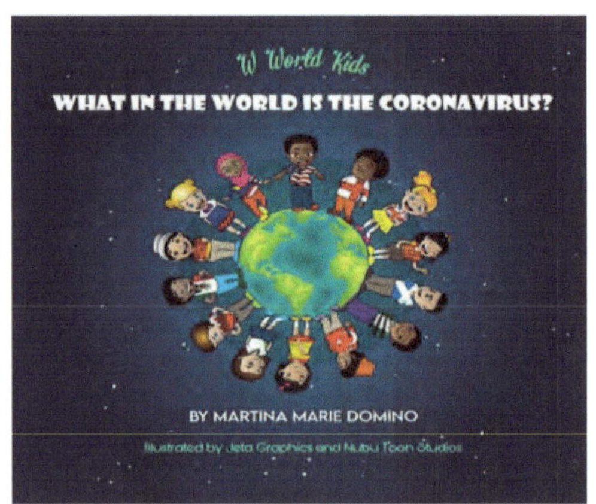

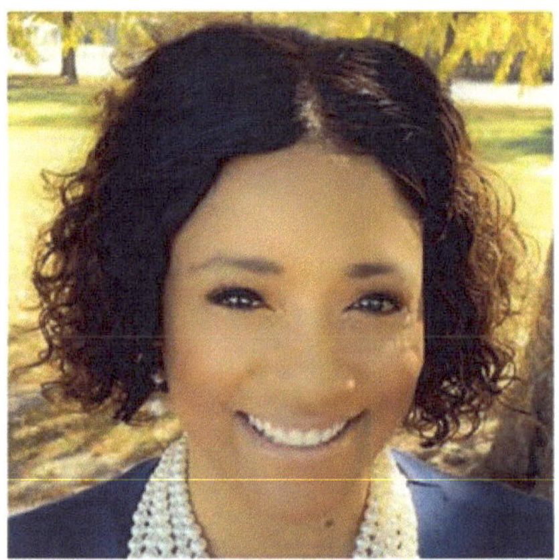

BOOK A VISIT WITH AUTHOR MARTINA DOMINO!

DESCRIPTION OF VIRTUAL SCHOOL PROGRAMS

STORIES (30 MINUTES)

This program is best for pre-K - 5th Grade. After sharing my book, "W World Kids, in the World is the Coronavirus ? ", I invite my listeners to explore the different ways we can protect ourselves from the coronavirus. Students will see and discuss face masks, hand sanitizer and other preventative measures to take to protect themselves during this pandemic.

Don't wait!

Book an in-person or virtual visit today!

TO BOOK A VISIT:

Simply fill out the author visit request form at:
www.martinadomino.com

When signing up, please be sure to mention who referred you/how you heard about the Author Visit program! !

STAY CONNECTED:

Instagram:
@authormartinadomino

Facebook:
@Martina Domino, Children's Author

MARTINADOMINO.COM